Radical Self-Care When You Are Ill

52 Skills and Affirmations to Help You Restore Your Well-Being

Debra Burdick

"I found many helpful ideas to guide myself into a better place. Dealing with chronic illness is hard, and these skills are a great tool. They can really help shift a bad day into a better one." Jennifer Lemieux.

"These skills always give me a different perspective when I put the suggestions they give me, into practice. Makes me feel a lot better." Lori N.

"This book, Radical Self Care When You Are Ill, is a lovely, gentle and supportive way to help. It teaches important skills that calm emotions; it also teaches new behaviors that can restore well-being." Shari Jackson.

Praise for Debra's Previous Books

Mindfulness for Kids with ADHD. "This wonderful, practical book is full of help and heart. Drawing on both sides of the brain, and integrating thinking and feeling, it has tons of specific suggestions and activities for kids and their parents. It's fun, to the point, encouraging, and hopeful. A real gem."—**Rick Hanson, PhD**, author of *Resilient*

Mindfulness for Teens with ADHD nails it! Any teen--indeed, any person--who has ADHD--indeed, any person, period--can gain enormously by using this practical, reader-friendly, immensely valuable workbook. I give this book the highest recommendation. It will reduce stress, build skills, and dramatically improve the life of every person who uses it." Edward **Hallowell, M.D.** Author of *Driven to Distraction*

Mindfulness Skills for Clinicians and Clients. Debra's work has changed my life as well as the lives of my patients. **Jose Colon, M.D., M.P.H.** Medical Director, Lee Health Sleep Center

ISBN: 9798878998512

Published by

The Brain Lady

Estero, FL

www.TheBrainLady.com

This book is dedicated to all those
who taught me that self-care is mandatory
to set the stage for healing.

Table of Contents

Introduction

Hello and welcome!

I am delighted that you are reading this book on your journey through physical or emotional illness. My intention and expectation is that you will find some specific skills and wisdom here that help you in a significant way to restore your physical, emotional and mind-body-spirit well-being. I hope that you will learn and use these skills to take the utmost care of yourself and set the stage for healing.

As a psychotherapist, award-winning author of five books and two card decks (Mindfulness Skills Workbook for Clinicians and Clients) and an international speaker I created and used the skills in this book (and card deck of the same name) originally to help myself deal with a chronic illness. I then used them to help other people deal with physical and emotional illness for over 30 years. You can learn more about my background and work at www.thebrainlady.com.

I have often been praised for my skill of translating the relevant research findings into easily accessible skills that help you get the benefits found by the studies. As you will soon see, my skills simply teach you how to do it!

My own 15 year journey through illness transformed me as a human and spiritual being. In the midst of my illness I prayed and promised God that when I got well I would write a book to help people who were dealing with illness in the hopes that using the skills I learned through my healing journey would make their journey much easier than mine had been.

God answered my prayers and I got well! This *Radical Self-Care When You Are Ill* book and the card deck of the same name fulfill the promise I made to God.

This book provides a radical approach to restoring your well-being and successfully coping with physical or emotional illness. Whether you're dealing with a chronic condition, recovering from surgery, or simply aiming to enhance your life despite health setbacks, this book offers essential skills to guide you.

You can use this collection of 52 skills and affirmations every day as a companion to your healing journey to navigate the challenges of illness and:

- Transform your healing journey and your life.

- Tap into the power of the mind and spirit to promote well-being.

- Thrive and live a good life despite feeling ill.

- Set the stage for healing.

- Restore a profound sense of well-being including physical, emotional and mind-body-spirit.

These skills are also designed to help you if you feel like you've tried everything but are still frustrated and discouraged as you deal with mysterious illness, chronic illness such as Fibromyalgia, arthritis, diabetes, or heart disease, mental health issues such as depression and anxiety as well as illness that has been deemed terminal.

Many of these skills are commonly used by those who experience radical remission of cancer as described in *Radical Remission: Surviving Cancer Against All Odds* by Kelly Turner.

Keep in mind that this book is not about illness. It is about restoring your well-being during and throughout illness. It is about thriving and living a good life despite feeling ill. It is about setting the stage for healing.

As mentioned earlier, this book was born out of my personal healing journey and my life's work as a psychotherapist, speaker and author. I had been ill with mysterious symptoms that doctors couldn't figure out, diagnose or effectively treat for more than 15 years. Eventually diagnosed with Fibromyalgia, Chronic Fatigue Syndrome, Leaky Gut and Chemical Sensitivities I found a variety of traditional and alternative treatments that gradually helped. Incorporating mindfulness and meditation into my daily life and learning about the power of our thoughts and divine connection in creating well-being were central components of my healing.

The skills provided in this book were learned the hard way through my own healing journey, from helping clients with illness (both physical and emotional) in my 25-year psychotherapy private practice, from teaching workshops and through constantly studying with leading experts and poring through the research on a wide variety of topics related to all aspects of healing. They are evidence-based, clinically tested skills you can use every day to learn and incorporate radical self-care to help you restore your physical, emotional and spiritual well-being when you are experiencing illness.

Thanks for being here! I wish you well from the bottom of my heart.

I love you!

Deb

About the Skills

This book provides a radical approach to successfully dealing with physical or emotional illness. It provides 52 skills and affirmations designed to help you restore all aspects of your well-being including physical, emotional and mind-body-spirit.

It includes wide ranging skills from the fields of Mindfulness, Cognitive Behavioral Therapy, Positive Psychology, Mind-Body Medicine and Spirituality as well as Affirmations for Healing to help restore well-being.

It also includes skills commonly used by those who experience radical remission of cancer.

Use the skills to help you get an accurate diagnosis, create a healing team, strengthen self-advocacy, and improve self-care and social support to foster healing.

Use the Mindfulness skills integrated throughout to engage the healing power of the mind-body connection.

Use the Mind-Body-Spirit skills to tap into your inner wisdom and the power of your spiritual beliefs and divine love and to enlist the aid of a higher power for healing.

For a digital card deck version of the skills visit

https://thebrainlady.com/radical-self-care-when-you-are-ill/

The skills presented in this book are not intended to substitute for the advice of your medical doctor or mental health professional.

Instructions and

Ideas for Use

You can use these radical self-care skills to help you restore your emotional, physical, and mind-body-spirit well-being. These skills help you examine your beliefs, make changes in your thought patterns, tame your emotions, and adopt new behaviors to take the best care of yourself so your well-being can be restored. These skills may also assist you in living a full life despite illness.

This book is divided into four sections.

- Emotional Self-Care

- Physical Self-Care

- Mind-Body-Spirit Self-Care

- Affirmations for Healing

Choose any skill, read it and do what it says. You can do this by yourself, with a friend or family member, or in a therapy session. You can use the skills anytime, before activities such as meals, work, or bedtime, or when you feel unwell or stressed to shift your mind and body into a healing place and reconnect with well-being.

Choose a time that works best for you and put it on your calendar or set an alarm to remind yourself to focus on the skill. As you gradually work through the skills notice how you are incorporating them into your daily life and how they are helping you restore your well-being.

Focus on one skill at a time. Read the skill aloud a couple of times and think about the skill for a few minutes. Then tune in to how you feel when you read it. Explore how the skill applies to you. Either do, or plan how and when to do, any action specified by the skill.

Pay attention to any resistance that comes up. Try to understand it and see if it is trying to tell you something. Acknowledge it, address it and then move forward. An example might be that you never seem to get around to writing down your answers on the worksheet. Or perhaps you read the skill but don't actually do it. Think about why not and how you can get yourself to move through the resistance and do what is needed to restore your well-being.

The more skills that you complete and incorporate into your life, the more progress you will make toward restoring your well-being.

Use the Radical Self-Care Worksheet provided at the end of the book to write down your answers when suggested. It will help you keep yourself organized and focused. It will also help you be accountable to yourself. When you have completed the skills, your worksheet will be a valuable reminder of the work you accomplished. You can download a copy of the worksheet **at https://thebrainlady.com/radical-self-care-downloads/** so you can print it out or download it to your computer. Then you can write on it or expand it in your word processor as you go through the skills.

If you are dealing with illness or treatments that impact your ability to concentrate and feel that writing answers on the worksheet is too difficult at this time, that's ok. Just do the skills as best you can.

Put a bookmark on the page of the skill you are working on and refer to it several times throughout the day and until you feel ready to move on to another skill.

If you choose a skill you have already done, notice how it feels to read it after having already done it or incorporating its message into your life. Pay attention to what, if anything, has changed since you first read the skill.

The link for the accompanying audio meditations for three of the skills is

https://thebrainlady.com/radical-self-care-downloads/

<<<<<+>>>>

Section One:

Emotional Self-Care

This section includes self-care skills that help you take care of your emotional health. They help you be more aware of how your illness is impacted by stress, your thought patterns, as well as your past, and then help you set your intention and shift your thoughts and feelings to promote well-being and healing.

Emotional Self-Care Skill 1.1

Set Your Intention

Setting your intention is the first step in accomplishing anything. What is your intention? What do you want to accomplish, especially related to restoring your well-being?

Do you intend to be completely healed? Do you intend to stay focused on positive thoughts and feelings that support your healing? Do you intend to get a better sleep routine and get more sleep? Do you intend to get help with your anxiety or depression? Do you intend to get more exercise? Do you intend to contact a specialist about your symptoms?

Create your own unique intention to feel well, restore your well-being and set the stage for your body and mind to heal. Write down your intention on the Radical Self-Care Worksheet and on a another paper and post it where you can see it daily to help you stay focused on your intention and repeatedly dismiss unhelpful thoughts and actions that distract you from your intention, whenever they arise

If it suits you, create your main intention and several lower-level intentions that support it. For example, if your main intention is to heal completely, a lower-level intention might be to eat a healing diet.

Set Your Intention

Set your intention to heal and to feel well. Be specific.

As soon as you notice you are focusing on how bad you feel or on unhelpful thoughts or actions bring your attention back to your intention to heal and to feel well.

Write down your healing intention and post it where you can see it every day.

Read it aloud every morning and evening.

Emotional Self-Care Skill 1.2

Ditch the Stress

Stress and particularly your response to stress impact the health of your mind and body. In fact, studies show that a large percentage of doctor visits are due to stress related illness.

Identify stressors in your life that may be negatively affecting your health and then find options for reducing these stressors whenever possible. For example, list 5 things that stress you. Then number them from most to least stressful. Then circle those that you can eliminate or reduce.

Now take the steps needed to ditch or reduce those that you circled. If a major stressor is your job, how can you change your current work situation or find a new one that is less stressful?

If you feel stressed by your illness, what would help you feel less stressed? Is there a way to ask for help when you feel too stressed?

Tune in to how you respond to stress and use options provided in this book for calming your mind and body and reducing your stress response.

Use the Radical Self-Care Worksheet at the end of the book to list and track the stressors you will change, avoid or eliminate.

Ditch the Stress

Be mindful of what stresses you.

Then whenever possible, change, reduce or eliminate the stressors.

Explore and then change how you respond to those stressors you cannot change.

Use the other skills in this book to calm your mind and body and turn down your stress response.

Emotional Self-Care Skill 1.3

Change the Channel

When we are ill it is not unusual to feel depressed, anxious, fearful, angry, helpless and hopeless. And it is often easy to become completely focused on our illness or our pain.

We now know that what we focus on and think about tends to increase in our life. This is exactly the opposite of what we want to attract and create in our life, especially when we are ill.

You can use The Change the Channel skill whenever you notice you are feeling bad either physically or emotionally, or both. This provides an effective way to change what you are thinking about to something that feels better and keeps your focus on positive self-care and healing.

What you are thinking about is the "channel" you are watching. Tune in throughout the day and notice what "channel" you tend to watch in your mind.

Pick three channels you could watch that would feel better to watch. Perhaps you could choose to watch your healthy, happy or calm channels.

Decide what you would put on each channel. Maybe you could put a nature scene on your calm channel such as a beautiful flower or the gentle waves at the beach. Maybe place an image of your child or grandchild on your happy channel. You get the idea.

Be specific and write them down on the Radical Self-Care Worksheet so you can refer to them when you need to change the channel in your mind.

Change the Channel

What channel are you watching in your mind?   Is it the happy, worry, sad, stressed out, illness or excited channel?

If it doesn't feel good to watch that channel, pretend to use an imaginary remote control to change the channel to one that feels better to watch.

If you are watching your worry channel, change to your calm channel. If you are watching your illness channel, change to your wellness channel.

What would you put on your channels that feel better to watch?

Emotional Self-Care Skill 1.4

What If?

Tune in to what would be different if you felt well and then imagine these changes have already happened. Doing so can help you shift into a healing mode. Set aside some time to think about what would be different in your life if you felt really well. Then make a list.

Perhaps you would be eating healthier, exercising more, or sleeping better. Maybe your pain would be gone or at least less. Perhaps you would have more energy. Maybe you would be able to work, at least part time. Maybe you would be having fun with friends. Maybe you would feel good most days and maybe even every day.

Now, with eyes closed, deeply imagine how you would **feel** if these things were already changed. Do this to reprogram your subconscious as you practice **feeling** how you would feel if these changes were done NOW.

Is there is any way to make a change to create any of the things you put on your list now despite feeling ill, no matter how small? For example, can you take a short walk, or rest to keep energy up, or talk with a friend?

This skill can be very helpful in helping you remember wellness. For some, it can initially create sadness as you realize the losses your illness has caused. It's ok, and often necessary, to get in touch with the loss in order to heal. Acknowledge it. Then gradually shift your thoughts to how it feels when you feel better.

What If?

What would be different in your life if you felt really well?

What if you were healthy, calm, clear, and positive?

Make a list of all the things that would be different in your life if you felt healed.

Then close your eyes and imagine that you are already healed. Be sure to imagine how you will feel when you are healed.

Emotional Self-Care Skill 1.5

What Needs to Change?

There can be many obstacles that get in the way of a person getting well. Perhaps you need to remove yourself from a toxic situation or relationship or job. Maybe you have difficulty eating healthy because you love sweets and keep them in the house where you cannot resist eating them. Or maybe you always try to do too much and are always stressed out.

Maybe you realize that your illness causes you to feel depressed or you are carrying trauma and you could use some help from a therapist.

Make a list things you know need to change in order for you to get well or even feel better. Use the Radical Self-Care Worksheet to help keep you organized.

Be specific. Even the smallest change can make a big difference.

Next, identify things on your list you can start changing right away. Then, mark the things that you need help with and list how you will get help.

Number them in order of priority and post your list where you can see it every day.

Notice how you feel after making each positive change.

What Needs to Change?

Make a list of things that need to change in order for you to get well or feel better.

Circle those that you can do starting today and number them in order of priority.

Post this list where you can see it every day.

Check things off when they are done and update your list regularly.

Emotional Self-Care Skill 1.6

Imagine Wellness

Our mind is a very powerful healer. By using your imagination you can practice feeling how you would feel if you felt well. Every time you do so you can send your body powerful healing messages.

Use this skill to explore how you would feel if you were well. Use your imagination to feel this way many times per day.

A key to success with this skill is to go beyond **thinking** about wellness and actually imagine how it **feels** in your mind and body.

You might be able to remember how you felt when you were well. If not, just imagine what you think it would feel like or how you want to feel.

Imagine Wellness

Close your eyes.

Imagine what it would feel like to be completely well.

What would you be thinking about?

What emotions would you feel?

How would your body feel?

Spend 20-30 seconds three times a day and a minute at bedtime imagining you are feeling completely well.

Make sure you imagine feeling it, not just thinking about it.

Emotional Self-Care Skill 1.7

Let It Go

Emotions play an integral part in the health of our body. Unhelpful emotions are stored in our body and are sometimes carried there for years without us realizing it. This is especially true for events that were traumatic to us. Then they may manifest as symptoms of illness in the body.

This skill prompts you to look within to see what you may be holding onto that no longer serves you. If you find this difficult or if it brings up unpleasant feelings or memories, you may want to work with a mental health professional to help you delve deeper into your stored emotions and release them.

A simple, but effective practice to help you let go of whatever needs to go is simply to imagine you are holding whatever you need to let go of in your hand. Then imagine it flying away like a butterfly. Just imagine letting it go. Let it go.

Then notice how you feel after doing this letting go process. Observe any feelings of relief, lightness, release, freedom.

Practice this as often as you need to let go of anything that no longer serves you.

Let It Go

What are you holding on to that you need to let go of?

What doesn't serve you anymore or makes you feel worse? What are you trying to control that you simply need to let go of? What anger, anxiety, sadness, resentment, disappointment or fear are you carrying in your body?

Imagine you are holding whatever needs to go in the palm of your hand. Open your hand and let it go much like a butterfly flying away. Let go of everything that needs to go.

Notice how you feel after doing so.

Notice what you are still holding onto.

Emotional Self-Care Skill 1.8

Mindfulness of Emotions

Emotions have a physical component that manifests in physical sensations in our body. This is how we typically recognize we are having an emotion. For example, our stomach hurts, our heart pounds, we feel hot, or perhaps our shoulders get tight.

First, tune in and identify what you are feeling in the present moment without judging or trying to change it. Name whatever the emotion is you notice.

Then spend a moment exploring where this emotion may be showing up in your body. For example, do you notice that your stomach hurts when you are anxious? Does your neck hurt when you are feeling stressed? Does your chest feel tight when you are angry? Have you noticed this feeling in your body before? Did you associate it with an emotion?

Is this a feeling you have felt it before? If so, what was going on then? How often do you feel this way?

Do you think this emotion is helpful or unhelpful to you? How do you think this emotion is impacting your illness?

Practice this periodically and especially when you are noticing a strong emotion.

Mindfulness of Emotion

Close your eyes. Take a deep breath and as you exhale tune in to your emotions.

Notice what you are feeling right now.

Name the feeling. Allow yourself to feel it without trying to change it.

Where does the feeling show up in your body? Have you felt this way before? Is it helpful or unhelpful?

Remember you have the feeling, the feeling is not who you are.

When you are ready open your eyes.

Practice this skill often to tune in and monitor your emotions and how they impact your body.

Emotional Self-Care Skill 1.9

Mindfulness of Thoughts

When we are ill it is easy for our thoughts to become focused on our symptoms or pain. When we tune into our thoughts we may discover a steady stream of unhelpful thoughts such as "I feel so bad today". "I hate feeling this way". "What if I don't get better?"

Daniel Amen explains his theory of Automatic Negative Thoughts (ANTs) in his book *Change Your Brain, Change Your Life.* ANTs are typically unhelpful thoughts we think over and over again that we probably don't realize we have.

First, focus on identifying your unhelpful ANTs. Pay attention to your thoughts and notice if they are helpful or unhelpful.

When you notice any automatic negative thoughts, then "exterminate the ANT" by finding a thought that you believe and that feels better when you think it. For example, you might replace the thought "I feel so bad today" with "Even though I feel bad today, I have felt better and I will take extra good care of myself today". Or, replace "I am so worried about my health" with "I do worry about my health but I am taking control of my health and have found a medical professional that I trust to help me."

Notice how you feel after exterminating the ANT.

Mindfulness of Thoughts

Tune in and notice what you are thinking about.

If the thought feels bad or is unhelpful, replace it with a thought that feels better and is believable.

For example: "I feel so bad today."

Replace it with "Even though I feel bad today, I have felt better and I will feel better again."

Emotional Self-Care Skill 1.10

Lazy River

Use the image of a lazy river common to most water parks to help you learn to dismiss unhelpful thoughts and to engage with helpful thoughts. Imagine you are watching rafts float by in a lazy river. Imagine some rafts are negative and some positive.

At first, just let the rafts go by and look upstream for the next one.

Now notice what the rafts carry. Let rafts go by if they carry pain, illness, or anything else that is stressful or negative. Just let them go by and look upstream to focus on the next raft.

After you have done this practice for a while, shift it a bit. When you notice a raft that is carrying something positive, fun, comforting or healing imagine getting in that raft and going for a ride as you stay focused on the positive feeling.

This process helps you practice letting pain, illness and negative thoughts go by without engaging in them so you can focus on positive, healing thoughts.

What rafts do you notice during the day? Practice focusing only on the positive ones and letting the others go by. Notice what changes in how you feel.

Have fun with this imagery.

Lazy River

Imagine you are watching colorful rafts float by in a lazy river like at a water park. Watch each raft as it goes by. Look upstream for the next one.

Imagine some rafts are negative or carrying pain or illness. Don't get in them, just let them go by.

Imagine some rafts are positive and full of healing and comfort. Get in one. Enjoy your healing ride down the lazy river.

Practice letting pain, illness and negative thoughts go by like the negative rafts so you can focus on positive, healing thoughts.

Emotional Self-Care Skill 1.11

Laugh

Norman Cousins demonstrated the power of laughter in his book *Anatomy of an Illness*. Laughter can be healing and most of us don't do it often enough.

Remember a time when you laughed out loud. Tune in to remember how you felt then.

Set your intention to notice funny things around you every day. What things make you smile or chuckle or laugh out loud? How can you have more of this in your life?

Practice laughing out loud every day. Let's start right now. Simply laugh. Ok, now laugh again. Now laugh and just keep laughing. Go for a true belly laugh.

How do you feel after laughing? Incorporate a good laugh into your day every day.

Laugh

Laughter can be healing.

Remember a time when you laughed out loud. Remember how you felt then.

Notice funny things around you:

- The funny antics of a child or pet
- A joke
- A comedy
- A pun or wordplay

Practice laughing out loud daily.

Just start laughing. Go ahead – laugh.

Keep laughing until it's hard to stop.

Emotional Self-Care Skill 1.12

Release the Past

Recent trauma research has shown that when we experience intense emotions due to any experience that feels traumatic to us, the emotions involved in our response to it can be stored in our cells. This often leads to physical and emotional illness. One of the things that many cancer patients who experienced radical remission did was explore and release these intense emotions from the past.

Make a list of past events that have caused strong negative emotions or that felt traumatic to you.

Do you think there is any correlation between when the past event occurred and the onset of your illness? For example did you develop heart disease after a loved one died? Did you get cancer or depression after a fire destroyed your home? Did you develop stomach problems when you had trouble letting go of your resentment about how badly your boss treated you? You get the idea.

If there is any possibility that a past experience might be contributing to your illness in the present, seek out a helping professional to help you do the more in-depth work that may be needed to process and release any remnants of these past emotions.

Release the Past

Make a list of past events that caused strong negative emotions.

Seek a helper who can guide you to release emotions that may be driving your subconscious in unhealthy ways and perhaps impacting your health.

Look online for some options that help:

- Psychotherapy
- Trauma Work
- EMDR
- EFT (Emotional Freedom Technique)
- Neurofeedback

Emotional Self-Care Skill 1.13

Secondary Gain

Hidden benefits occur when a person who is ill experiences some type of hidden benefit, often called secondary gain, due to being ill. For example, their illness might serve as a great excuse to stay home when they don't want to take part in a difficult family gathering or go to a toxic work environment. They might get out of taking care of others when they are ill which relieves their guilt. They may get others to do things for them that they might be capable of doing for themselves. They may use the illness to excuse a pattern of not managing their emotions.

This is often driven from deeply hidden unconscious issues that they are not aware of. When they do get a hidden benefit from being ill they will lose that benefit if they get well. This can keep some people stuck in illness.

Look at what hidden benefits being ill might provide for you, both intentional and subconscious. Ask your family and friends if they see you using your illness as an excuse.

It's often necessary to ask for help but you must confront the fact that you may need to give up these hidden benefits and find healthier options for dealing with difficult issues in order to get better.

Secondary Gain

Think about how you might be using your illness to get a secondary gain.

For example, do you use illness as an excuse to get out of doing things, or to get others to do things for you that you could do for yourself, or do you expect special treatment?

Be honest with yourself.

It's often necessary to ask for help but be mindful of how you might have developed a pattern of using your illness as an excuse.

You must give up this behavior to be well.

<<<<+>>>>

Section Two: Physical Self-Care

This section includes self-care skills that help you take care of your physical health. This includes dealing effectively with the medical community; gathering a positive healing team; coping with and shifting pain; eating, sleeping and moving to take extreme care of yourself; resting when you are tired and using mindfulness and nature to help your body relax to foster healing.

Physical Self-Care Skill 2.1

Working with the Medical Community

It can be challenging to discuss your symptoms and feel like your concerns are taken seriously when dealing with some members of the medical community. Studies show that the more questions you ask your medical provider the better your outcome is likely to be. Therefore, it can be essential to your care to prepare questions for each visit.

Also, do your research before each visit. This should include looking at any bloodwork or medical testing you have had done and highlighting what has changed or is flagged as out of norm so you can ask the provider about it. Also, it can help to look online for medical research that studies the treatments for your symptoms/diagnosis. Ask your provider for educational materials about your illness. The more informed you are the better questions you can ask and the better care you will receive.

Be sure to find providers that welcome your questions and are willing to discuss things with you. Some people even interview prospective medical providers to be sure they are a good fit. Keep in mind that some providers are more open to questions than others.

It is imperative that you take control of your health to get a better outcome. This skill helps you do just that.

Working with the Medical Community

Research shows that if you ask lots of questions you will have a better outcome.

Make a list of questions to ask your doctor.

Ask for explanations. Be sure you understand the reasoning, and the research behind and possible side effects of treatment and medications.

If you feel your provider discounts your concerns or doesn't listen, find another provider.

Physical Self-Care Skill 2.2

Get an Accurate Diagnosis

In order to get proper treatment one must first get an accurate diagnosis. Getting an accurate diagnosis can often involve a number of diagnostic tests and consulting an array of medical providers. Sometimes this can be a multi-step process and is often frustrating, time consuming and frightening.

When you receive a diagnosis make sure the diagnosis you have been given makes sense to you. Remember, you must take control of your health so ask questions and do your research and learn about possible diagnosis for your symptoms.

Consult with your medical provider and consider the possibility that you may need to get a second or maybe even a third opinion. In order to get an accurate diagnosis (and thus, proper treatment) you may need to visit a major medical center that specializes in symptoms like yours.

Get an Accurate Diagnosis

In order to get the proper treatment you must have an accurate diagnosis.

Make sure the diagnosis makes sense to you. Get a second, third or maybe even a fourth opinion if needed.

Seek a provider who specializes in your symptoms and diagnosis.

Visit a major medical center that treats your illness even if it requires you to travel.

Physical Self-Care Skill 2.3

Gather Your Healing Team

A healing team is extremely supportive to your healing journey and dealing successfully with illness. Many types of members belong on your team such as medical providers, mental health providers, alternative healers, religious or spiritual members, family, friends, nature and even pets.

You will gather your own unique collection of people who will encourage you, guide you, love you and in many different ways, take care of you. Be careful to select the best people to be on your healing team.

Think about what you need and how each person contributes to your healing. Be specific and ask for what you need from each member.

List your healing team members on your Radical Self-Care Worksheet including their contact information. Be prepared to add additional members and sometimes let members go as you progress and your needs change.

Gather Your
Healing Team

Make a list on the worksheet of who belongs on your healing team.

Allow only those who are honest, helpful, validating, encouraging, knowledgeable, inspiring and positive and who can see you well again.

Team members can be from various sources such as medical, mental health, alternative healers, religious or spiritual, family, friends, and even pets.

Be clear about what you need from each member and how they support your well-being.

Physical Self-Care Skill 2.4

Advocate for Yourself

You've heard the saying 'the squeaky wheel gets the oil''. Studies show that people who ask their health care providers questions and demand clear explanations of symptoms and treatments get well faster and more often that those who do not.

You will have a better outcome if you take control of your health. Advocating for yourself is one important part of doing so. Self-advocacy empowers you and promotes active involvement and shared decision-making.

The first step is finding a medical or alternative provider that you can trust and that is open and willing to answer your questions. Advocating for yourself includes being prepared, taking notes, speaking up about your concerns, getting your questions answered, feeling heard and getting what you need.

If you cannot advocate for yourself then ask someone to do it for you. This can be a family member, a friend or even a professional health advocate.

Advocate for Yourself

Ask for what you need.

Be a squeaky wheel to get your needs met.

Do your homework.

Look up your symptoms and treatment options.

Ask questions.

Keep records.

Ask for someone to advocate for you if you are not able such as family, a friend or even a professional health advocate if needed.

Physical Self-Care Skill 2.5

Eat to Heal

Food can be thought of as a form of natural medicine. But some foods can be detrimental to your health.

Many who experienced radical remission from cancer radically changed their diet. Learn about what foods support your healing and which do not. At a minimum make sure you stay hydrated, limit sugar and unhealthy fats, and eat lots of plant based foods. Choose organic foods to avoid toxins such as pesticides, hormones, antibiotics and food additives. And keep your weight in normal ranges.

Consider meeting with a Nutritionist who specializes in helping people with your symptoms to give you the components of a healing diet.

Be mindful of what you eat and ask yourself if each bite you take is helping you heal. Even making small micro changes can add up to give you a powerful boost in healing.

Write down changes you plan to make to your diet to support healing on the Radical Self-Care Worksheet.

Eat to Heal

Be mindful to make sure that everything you put into your mouth supports your health.

Ask yourself "Will this food help me heal?"

Stay hydrated.

Avoid sugar and unhealthy fats.

Eat organic food to avoid toxins.

Eat only what you need to maintain a healthy weight.

Keep a food diary to track what foods increase or decrease symptoms.

Consider a plant-based or mostly plant-based lifestyle.

Find herbs or supplements that support your health.

Physical Self-Care Skill 2.6

Sleep to Heal

The body and mind require sleep to stay healthy and especially to heal when ill. Start thinking about sleep as a form of medicine and give getting a good night's sleep top priority.

Figure out how much sleep makes you feel the best by keeping track of how you feel on days after you didn't sleep well compared to days when you got a good night's sleep. Then set your sleep schedule to accommodate the ideal amount for you. Most adults do best with 7-9 hours per night. But everyone is different. Keep in mind that studies show that sleeping too much can make you feel as bad as too little sleep. Write how much sleep serves you best and when you will go to bed and when you will get up on the Radical Self-Care Worksheet.

Follow the guidelines for good sleep hygiene to set yourself up to get the best sleep. These guidelines include going to bed and getting up at the same time every day, even on weekends. Sleep is very habitual. So be mindful to follow the same schedule every day, even on the weekends.

Set up your bedroom for sleep (and maybe sex) and Nothing Else. Get rid of work, computers, TVs, cell phones, hobbies, laundry, etc. Make sure your bed is truly comfortable. Stop drinking caffeine by mid-afternoon if it keeps you awake. Stop drinking all liquids after dinner if they make you often have to get up to pee. Avoid screens for an hour before bed. Set the temperature to a cool temperature to promote better sleep, and avoid lights and noise.

Sleep to Heal

Think of sleep as a form of medicine.

Figure out how much sleep makes you feel the best. Write it on the worksheet.

Go to sleep and get up at the same time every day. Write it on the worksheet.

Avoid screens, sugar, caffeine and activating shows or books before bedtime.

Set up the bedroom for sleep (& sex) and Nothing Else.

Get a comfortable, supportive bed. Set the temperature a bit cool. Block out all sound and light.

Consult a sleep specialist to rule out sleep apnea and for natural sleep aids if needed.

Physical Self-Care Skill 2.7

Keep Moving

The human body is designed to move. Although illness can impair your ability to move it is essential to keep moving within the limits of your illness. The myriad benefits of moving your body include flexibility, muscle strength, circulation, mood, sleep, pain, immune function and weight and so much more!

Figure out what movement you are capable of and that you enjoy. If you cannot do an exercise such as Yoga on the floor, then do it in a chair. If you can't walk for 10 minutes then walk for 1 minute. Use a cane or walker to help you balance. If you can't walk at all, then stretch your arms, legs, neck and shoulders while seated, or even lying down. Just MOVE!

Start slowly and gradually increase intensity and duration as your illness allows. Be careful not to overdo or to push yourself too fast.

Plan to incorporate movement in your life and make a commitment to moving every day. Schedule regular exercise and put it on your calendar. Write what you will do and when on the Radical Self-Care Worksheet.

Keep Moving

Moving your body any way you are able is essential to healing.

Moving improves mood, sleep, weight, strength, flexibility and pain.

Do whatever exercise you enjoy.

Start as small as tolerated and gradually increase intensity and duration.

Aim for at least 30 minutes 3-4 times per week even if it's simply stretching, taking a walk or doing chair exercises.

Write down how you will incorporate moving into your daily life and put a reminder on your calendar.

Physical Self-Care Skill 2.8

Shift the Pain

Pain can be overwhelming and often significantly interferes with your quality of life. Pain can easily become so intense that you can hardly think about anything else. What you focus on tends to increase, so the more you think about pain, the more pain you are likely to feel.

Use the following 4-step process to help you acknowledge and embrace your pain and then gently shift your attention away from the pain whenever you need a break from it.

Do this periodically whenever you have pain.

It is extremely important to treat pain and not let it get out of control. Be sure to discuss options for pain management with your medical team.

Shift the Pain

Notice where you have pain in your body and/or mind.

Bring your attention to the center of the pain.

Now move your attention slowly to the edges of the pain.

Shift your focus away from the pain by paying attention to an area of your body or mind that feels comfortable.

Now touch your forefinger to the tip of your thumb and stay focused there until you notice your pain has eased a bit.

Repeat several times a day or when you want a brief break from pain.

Physical Self-Care Skill 2.9

Set Mindful Limits

It can be difficult to accept that illness often puts limits on what you are able to accomplish. Think about how you feel when you do too much or feel stressed out because you have so many demands on you. Tune in to how your illness is impacted by stress or when you overdo.

Spend some time thinking about how you can set healthy limits on what you try to do. Maybe you can look at all the things on your to-do list and start taking things off the list that could be done by someone else, or that are not totally necessary. For example, perhaps you can ask an adult child to mop the kitchen floor or hire a cleaning crew rather than doing it yourself and exhausting yourself.

It's important that you step back and look at what you can reasonably expect of yourself while you are ill. How does your illness limit you? It works better to reduce your load and rest when you are tired, rather than trying to overdo and then relapse into exhaustion and increased symptoms for the next few days.

Honor your limits to take the best care of yourself. You can expand them if your illness allows. But even then avoid overdoing it to prevent worsening of your symptoms.

Set Mindful Limits

Think about how you feel when you overdo or do too much.

How can you set reasonable limits on what you try to accomplish at any given time to avoid feeling exhausted, stressed or increased pain?

How can you be kind to yourself and make guilt-free resting an integral part of your healing journey?

Honor your limits to take care of yourself and allow yourself to heal.

Physical Self-Care Skill 2.10

Remember Wellness

Dr. Herbert Benson, a renowned Harvard cardiologist explains the concept of "Remembered Wellness" in his book by that name. He discovered that a certain percentage of people who participate in studies and who receive a placebo instead of the actual treatment, get well, even though they didn't receive the treatment, but believed they did. In fact the placebo effect is so powerful that all studies need to account for its presence to make sure the effect of the treatment being studied is larger than the placebo effect. Dr. Benson went on to recommend that the placebo effect be renamed "remembered wellness".

Our thoughts and beliefs can have a significant impact on our bodies. One study showed that people who spent time imagining they were exercising actually got stronger without exercising!

The theory for this Remember Wellness skill is to remember a time when you felt really well. Your mind doesn't know the difference between current reality and what you are imagining and it can recreate what you are remembering and manifest that remembered wellness in your body. If you cannot remember feeling well, then imagine what it would feel like.

If this skill puts you in touch with the losses illness has caused, accept and acknowledge your feelings, then gradually shift to remembering or imagining wellness. Listen to a longer audio version of this meditation at https://thebrainlady.com/radical-self-care-downloads/.

Remember Wellness

Close your eyes and remember a time when you felt well (or imagine it if you can't remember).

Remember how you felt then and imagine you feel that way now.

Remember or imagine how your body feels good and your mind is positive and content.

Bring that feeling into the present.

Imagine a sense of profound well-being.

Practice this repeatedly throughout the day until it becomes an automatic habit.

Listen to a longer audio version of this meditation online.

Physical Self-Care Skill 2.11

Relax Your Body

Dr. Edmund Jacobsen discovered that tightening a muscle and holding the tension for 7-10 seconds and then releasing the tension for at least 10 seconds resulted in the muscle being less tense. This technique can be extremely helpful to release tension that is being triggered by pain.

Use this skill to do a progressive relaxation of the major muscle groups in your body using the technique used in Dr. Jacobsen's research. The result will be a feeling of physical relaxation and decreased pain - and more importantly, an overall decrease in your stress response.

Practice this skill daily and notice what has changed in your mind and body each time you are finished.

Listen to a longer audio version of the meditation at https://thebrainlady.com/radical-self-care-downloads/.

Relax Your Body

Tighten your hands and fingers into a fist and hold for 7 seconds.

Release them for 10 seconds.

Tighten your face including eyes, cheeks and mouth by scrunching into a tight smile and hold for 7 seconds.

Release for 10 seconds.

Repeat this tightening and releasing process with your chest, shoulders, feet, legs, back, belly.

Notice the difference between how a tight versus relaxed muscle feels.

Notice what has shifted in your mind and body as this practice relaxes your mind and body.

Listen to the audio version.

Physical Self-Care Skill 2.12

Body Scan

Jon Kabat Zinn created a meditation process called a Body Scan to progressively tune into each area of the body and notice what is there. The benefits of using this process include physical and emotional calming, as well as increased awareness of how the body is impacted by emotions such as stress and anxiety.

As you do this meditation, tune in to how each part of your body feels. Just notice what's there without trying to change it. Is that part of your body, tense, relaxed, warm, cold, energized, tired, aching, or perhaps comfortable?

Emotions almost always have a physical component that shows up in your body. Pay attention to what emotions you may have been experiencing that are showing up as tension or discomfort in various parts of your body.

With practice you will be able to use physical sensations as a key to emotions. For example, do you get a stomachache when you are nervous or worried? Do you get a stiff or sore neck when you feel stressed?

Practice a slow Body Scan every day. When you have practiced it slowly for a few days and feel comfortable doing it, then you can also do a quick Body Scan whenever you have a moment when you are feeling stressed out.

Run through the Body Scan at least once a day. Enjoy being able to calm your mind and relax your body. This is a great antidote to stress as it quickly gets you out of your head and calms your stress response.

Body Scan

Bring your attention to your body.

Pay attention to your feet.

Notice everything there is to notice about your legs.

Move up to your hips and bottom.

Bring your attention to your belly and chest.

Move up through your back and on up to your neck and head.

Notice your hands and arms.

Let go of anything in your body that you don't need. Let it go.

How does your body feel now that you have paid attention to it?

Remember, your attention is calming and healing.

Physical Self-Care Skill 2.13

Rest When You Are Tired

Like most people, you probably have many things to get done and your responsibilities don't magically disappear when you are ill. You may find that you push yourself to get things done even though you are feeling tired or even exhausted. When you just keep going and don't rest when you are tired you may discover that you become significantly more exhausted and that your symptoms get worse or at a minimum don't improve.

Also, sometimes when you feel a little better you may do even more and then find that you did too much and then feel exhausted. And then your symptoms may worsen as well. When you do this you may create a vicious cycle of extreme ups and downs in both your energy and symptoms.

Instead, if you tune into your energy level and match your energy output to the energy you have at the moment and pace yourself if you feel better than usual, you may find your energy and your symptoms remain more stable.

Print out "I Rest When I am Tired" and post it where you can see it to remind you.

Incorporate this skill into every day as soon as possible and Rest When You Are Tired. Doing this can support healing and improve well-being.

Rest When
You are Tired

Periodically tune into your energy level. When it is low or waning, take a break and rest.

Set an alarm to remind you to check in with yourself so you can rest before you become exhausted.

Repeat out loud:

"I rest when I am tired."

Notice how your energy level evens out when you rest before you are worn out.

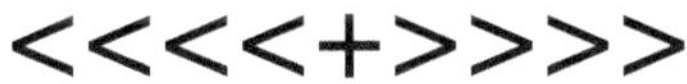

Section Three:

Mind-Body-Spirit Self-Care

This section includes self-care skills that help you take care of your mind-body-spirit (m-b-s) connection. One skill helps you find ways to be of service to others; another to strengthen your social support system; and another to solidly define your reasons for getting well.

Other skills in this section help you tap into the power of your spiritual beliefs and divine love to enlist the aid of a higher power to access unconditional love and healing,

Most of these skills were commonly done by people who experienced radical remission from cancer.

M-B-S Self-Care Skill 3.1

I Believe

Dr. Kelly Turner, author of *Radical Remission* found that one of the things that people who experienced radical remission from cancer did was to deepen their spiritual connection to some sort of spiritual energy, daily, in order to receive its healing benefits.

This Mind-Body-Spirit self-care skill encourages you to take the first step and think about what you believe in whether it is God, a higher power, the Divine, inner wisdom, infinite intelligence, a particular religious doctrine, spiritual energy or even no religious or spiritual belief.

Write down what you believe in on the Radical Self-Care Worksheet and how you can use your religious or spiritual beliefs and spiritual energy to support your well-being and healing. Think about times in the past when your spiritual beliefs have helped you.

I Believe

What do you believe?

For example, do you believe in:

- God
- Higher power
- Infinite intelligence
- Source
- Inner being
- Divine
- Universe
- Inner Wisdom
- Spiritual Energy
- Other?

How can you tap into your religious or spiritual beliefs to support your healing and well-being?

Write down your answer.

M-B-S Self-Care Skill 3.2

Let Unconditional Love Flow

Anita Moorjani experienced a near death experience. In her book *Dying to Be Me*, she explains that during this experience she learned that we all have a steady stream of unconditional divine love that is available to us at all times. She states that this love is powerfully healing. She notes that unfortunately we can block its flow through our beliefs, thoughts, habits, fear and stress response.

This Mind-Body-Spirit self-care skill helps you tune into this flow of love and dissolve obstructions that restrict or prevent its flow. Spend a few moments thinking about a time when you felt loved and totally accepted for who you are. If you cannot think of such a time, imagine how that would feel.

As you do this skill, think of stresses in your life, limiting beliefs, fears or negative thoughts that may prevent unconditional love from flowing through you. Perhaps you harbor some type of resentment, you don't feel good enough or worthy of love, you are carrying the remnants of trauma in your cells, you feel angry or victimized, or you are fearful and anxious.

Visualize any obstructions simply dissolving as the unconditional love flows freely through you. If you struggle to allow them to dissolve consider working with a mental health professional to help you clear them.

Do this visualization many times each day.

Listen to a longer audio version of this meditation at
https://thebrainlady.com/radical-self-care-downloads/

____

Let Unconditional Love Flow

Imagine a wide pathway from above through which divine unconditional love that is available to everyone is flowing freely into your mind and body.

Give the flowing love a color.

Imagine any obstructions to the flow gently dissolving.

Let it flow.

Feel the warmth as you allow this love to fill and heal you.

Send your own unconditional love to your mind and body to take extreme care of yourself.

Listen to a longer audio version of this at https://thebrainlady.com/radical-self-care-downloads/

____

M-B-S Self-Care Skill 3.3

Ask For Help

Many people find it difficult to ask anyone for help. Keep in mind that everyone needs help sometimes and during illness it is particularly important to ask for the help you need. Most people want to help and are glad to help with specific things.

This self-care skill involves asking for help on 2 levels. On the first level it guides you to identify what you need help with in your healing journey. Then it asks you to make a list of who you can ask for help. Remember to include your healing team and family on your list.

Then, on the second level this skill prompts you to tune in to your higher power and ask for what you need. An important part of this is to thank your higher power as if you have already received the help. And then tune in to how you will feel when help has been given.

Despite having a religious or spiritual framework, many people are uncomfortable or not familiar with tuning in to their higher power to ask for help. Give it a try!

Ask for Help

What do you need help with?

Make a list of who you can ask for help.

Ask for help when you need it. Be specific.

Now tune into your personal version of your higher power.

Ask for help when you need it to restore your well-being.

Be specific.

Say "thank you" as if you have already received help.

Imagine feeling how you will feel when you receive help.

Tune in and watch for the help to arrive.

M-B-S Self-Care Skill 3.4

Connect To the Earth

This Mind-Body-Spirit self-care skill is based on the findings of recent studies that show that being physically in contact with the earth grounds us electrically and can reduce inflammation in the body. Other research suggests that simply being outside in nature can be healing.

Go outside regularly and use this skill to tap into the win-win benefits of grounding and of being in nature.

Notice what changes in your mind and body as you immerse yourself in nature while being connected to the earth.

Connect to the Earth

Find a place to sit outside where your bare feet can touch the earth or grass for about 20 minutes.

Take a deep breath and pay attention to what you can see, hear, smell and touch while you are outside, being still and connected to the earth.

Notice how you feel before and after doing this practice.

What, if anything, has changed in your mind or body?

Do this at least several times per week.

M-B-S Self-Care Skill 3.5

Healing Prayer

Although the effectiveness of prayer for healing has been hard to study scientifically, it has been found to be extremely powerful over the ages. One study showed improvements in depression and anxiety after praying. Some researchers think prayer conveys many of the same benefits as meditation.

Prayer transcends the human condition. When you use the power of prayer for healing during illness you may experience many benefits including calmness, peace, faith, hope and positivity. Many have reported they experienced healing from prayer, including spontaneous remission.

This skill provides a simple but effective prayer you can use to pray for healing. Try it out and see how it feels to you.

Then write your own version of a healing prayer that aligns with your personal beliefs. Use the Radical Self-Care Worksheet. Express praise, and gratitude along with your petition for healing (or what you are praying for). Notice how you feel before and after praying.

Look for evidence in your life that prayer is working for you.

Healing Prayer

Pray and ask for divine love and healing. For example:

"Lord God/Goddess of my being,

Unto the Father/Mother within;

Send your divine love into my mind and body.

Clear all obstructions to allow your unconditional love to flow and to fill my body, mind and spirit and heal me effortlessly and completely.

Thank you for your divine love and healing."

Write your own personal healing prayer asking for love and healing.

M-B-S Self-Care Skill 3.6

Healing Meditation

Meditation has been shown to be effective for reducing stress, anxiety, depression, pain and more. This skill uses the power of the mind and visualization for healing. It provides a healing meditation based on a healing white light that is often part of spiritual healing techniques.

Imagine a white, healing light flowing throughout your body. The aim is to set the stage for healing.

Notice how you feel before and after doing this meditation. What has changed?

Repeat this meditation regularly.

____

Healing Meditation

Close your eyes and imagine a bright healing light shining into the top of your head.

Imagine this light is lighting up and healing all the areas of your brain.

Watch as the light gradually fills your whole body starting from your head, down your spine, into your torso, legs and out through the bottoms of your feet.

Feel the warmth of the light as it continues to flow replacing any darkness with healing energy.

Allow yourself to let go of anything you simply don't need as the light cleanses and heals your body.

_______________.

M-B-S Self-Care Skill 3.7

Healing Images

Find or create an image that represents healing to you. Search images online or take a photo of something you find healing. Look at sample images until you find one that evokes a calm feeling of well-being.

Everyone is different but some examples might be a photo of a flower, a calm lake, a peaceful scene from the countryside, a photo of a child or grandchild, a photo of you when you were well, or of an activity that you will do when you feel good.

Place a picture of your healing image where you can see it every day to help you stay focused on healing instead of illness.

———————————

Healing Images

Find or create an image that represents healing to you:

Close your eyes and ask your higher power to give you a healing image that represents divine wellness.

Search for "healing images" on the internet and find one that resonates with you.

Think of symbols or images in your life that may already represent healing to you.

Place a picture of your healing image where you can see it every day to help you stay focused on healing instead of illness.

———————————

M-B-S Self-Care Skill 3.8

Ask For Guidance

Use this guided meditation to help you go within and ask for whatever guidance or wisdom you need right now. Picture the image of a blank white board and wait for answers to appear on the board. Answers may appear in words or pictures or symbols. Some people have received important messages that helped them heal in various ways.

Practice this skill and use it whenever you feel stuck or when you need guidance on what to do next.

Write down the guidance you receive on the <u>Radical Self-Care Worksheet</u> and refer back to it often.

Ask for Guidance

Close your eyes.

Take a deep breath and then exhale slowly through pursed lips.

Imagine a blank white board.

Ask for whatever guidance or wisdom you need right now.

Wait quietly for the answer to appear on the white board either in text or a picture or a symbol.

When you notice your mind has wandered (and it will) just bring it back to the white board over and over again.

Open your eyes and write down the guidance you received.

M-B-S Self-Care Skill 3.9

Tune In To Loved Ones

When people are asked if they have ever had any form of communication with their loved ones in spirit, most will answer, "Yes" and tell you what they experienced. This often occurs whether they were looking for it or not. This communication can take many forms.

Use the process in this skill to deliberately connect with loved ones who are in spirit to ask for support in healing or whatever you need to know.

Be patient and look for answers that may appear in various forms.

Practice doing this skill to improve your ability to receive answers.

Write down what you receive on the Radical Self-Care Worksheet and add to it each time you do this skill. Refer back to what you have received over time.

Tune in to Loved Ones

Close your eyes and picture a loved one who is now in spirit.

See their face in your mind and greet them.

Ask them what you need to know or do to support your healing.

Be specific.

Breathe slowly and patiently as you await their response.

Look for words, a picture, a feeling, a sound, a smell, a symbol, a knowing – anything that represents their answer.

Write down what you received.

M-B-S Self-Care Skill 3.10

My Reasons

Studies show that having a compelling reason or reasons to get well can contribute to healing. This Mind-Body-Spirit self-care skill guides you to get in touch with your unique and compelling reason(s) to get well by answering the questions "Why do I want to be well and be alive?" and "What will be different when I am well?"

Think about what motivates you to do what you need to do to heal. What brings joy, happiness and meaning to your life? What has your illness restricted you from doing that you love to do, and you want to do again? Do you want to dance like you used to? Do you want to attend your granddaughter's wedding? Do you want to enjoy more quality time with your spouse? Do you want to write that book that's been running through your mind? Do you have something you want to share with the world? Do you simply want to feel healthy and vibrant?

Write down your answer in the Radical Self-Care Worksheet and also post it where you can see it every day.

Use this skill in conjunction with Affirmation 4-13. After defining your reasons and using the Affirmation for a couple of days, what changed? Did you notice any change in your attitude or mood? Did you see any difference in your motivation to take care of yourself? What emotions arose as you connected to your reasons to get well? Did you feel sad about the losses your illness has caused such as not being able to do things you used to do? Did any of your initial reasons change?

My Reasons

Make a list of compelling reasons why you want to be well and why you want to live.

Answer the questions:

- "Why do I want to be well and be alive?"
- "What will be different when I am well?"

Post this list where you can see it every day.

M-B-S Self-Care Skill 3.11

Intuition/Inner Wisdom

Intuition is the ability to obtain direct knowledge about something without thinking. You know that gut feeling you get about something, or a sense of knowing that something is going to happen. It is that intangible information that spontaneously shows up in a feeling, a sense, a knowing, without mental thought. It comes from our subconscious rather than our conscious thought.

Often, our intuition is amazingly accurate, especially about our health. Therefore it can be helpful to deliberately tune into our intuition.

Use the meditation provided in this skill to help you tap into your intuition or inner wisdom to ask for guidance. Look for the information to be presented in various ways including a sense, a feeling, a knowing, an image, or even a symbol.

Practice this skill regularly to get better at accessing your intuition.

Also, notice when you get an intuitive nudge throughout your day and pay attention to how accurate it is. The more you tune into your intuition, the more information you will get and the greater the accuracy is likely to be.

Be sure to write down what you receive on the Radical Self-Care Worksheet.

Intuition/Inner Wisdom

Close your eyes and imagine you are sitting in a beautiful garden.

Be still and breathe in through your nose and slowly out through your mouth.

Set your intention to connect with your intuition.

Ask for guidance. Ask for signs that help you communicate with your inner wisdom and intuition.

Then relax and just be. Wait, watch and listen to what is presenting itself to you.

Trust that you are receiving exactly what you need to know right now.

Open your eyes when you are ready and write down the wisdom you received.

M-B-S Self-Care Skill 3.12

Be of Service

Studies show that helping others can promote a sense of well-being and healing. It can also reduce an unhealthy tendency to become too focused on illness.

Use this Mind-Body-Spirit self-care skill to explore ways to be of service to others within the limits of your illness and without exhausting yourself. Find ways to help that use your expertise and that you enjoy doing. Be careful to avoid situations that feel stressful. Write down how you will be of service on the Radical Self-Care Worksheet.

Be of Service

Find a way, no matter how small, to be of service to someone.

Perhaps you could:

- ✓ Volunteer at a favorite charity or school or church or…
- ✓ Help or encourage others dealing with illness
- ✓ Write about your journey
- ✓ Share your knowledge
- ✓ Telephone a friend or family
- ✓ Care for a pet
- ✓ Answer a help line
- ✓ Knit prayer shawls
- ✓ Look up ways to help others

Notice how you feel when you know you have helped someone.

Be careful not to overdo it.

Write down how your will be of service on the Worksheet.

M-B-S Self-Care Skill 3.13

Social Support

Being ill can be a very lonely experience. Studies show that those with a good social support system fare better emotionally and physically than those without one a good support system.

This Mind-Body-Spirit self-care skill guides you to identify your current social support system and then to explore options for expanding it if needed.

Think about how your current social support system works for you and how it meets your needs. List your support system on the <u>Radical Self-Care Worksheet</u>. Then explore options for making it work better for you and to expand it if you need more support. Write down how your will expand your support system on the <u>Radical Self-Care Worksheet</u>.

Aim for building a social support system that not only meets your various needs but that also helps your feel loved and cared about.

Social Support

Who is part of your social support system?

How can you enlarge your social support system if needed?

Where can you expand your interests and meet more like-minded people? Perhaps do a search online for groups that share your interests.

Where can you find a community of others dealing with the same illness in person or online?

What do you need to do differently to make your social support system work better for you?

Make a list of your current support system that works well.

Make a list of potential sources of support.

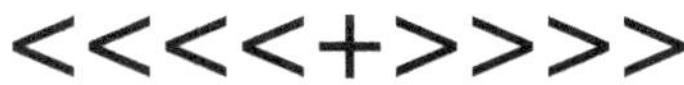

Section Four:

Mindful Affirmations for Healing

This section contains thirteen Affirmations you can use regularly to practice shifting mindset, emotions and behavior and to keep you laser focused on your self-care to help you restore your well-being. Each Affirmation is a powerful way to reinforce and consolidate the skills in the rest of the book.

Each affirmation explains why it's useful. Practice them regularly and incorporate them into your daily life.

Notice what changes in your life as you incorporate the Affirmations into your day.

Self-Care Affirmation 4.1

I Am Getting Well

This affirmation helps you rewire your brain for healing by repeating an affirmation that focuses on getting well, having everything you need to heal, and remembering how it feels to feel well.

===============

I am Getting Well

Repeat the following out loud many times during the day. Do your best to ignore any doubt that pops up.

> **"I am getting well.**
>
> **My mind and body have everything they need to heal.**
>
> **I am feeling better and better.**
>
> **I love how I feel when I am well.**
>
> **I am remembering how I feel when I am completely well."**

===============

Self-Care Affirmation 4.2

That Feels Better

This affirmation reminds you to find a thought that feels better when you feel bad. Practice it regularly and soon you will notice having more positive thoughts than negative.

===============

That Feels Better

Repeat the following.

"When I feel bad,

I will feel better when

I find a thought

that feels better."

Practice finding a thought that feels better throughout your day.

===============

Self-Care Affirmation 4.3

I Do What I Need To

This affirmation helps you stay focused on doing whatever Self-Care skills you need to support your well-being.

===============

I Do What I Need To

Repeat this out loud several times a day to help you stay focused on creating well-being:

"I do whatever

Self-Care skills I need to do

to support my well-being."

===============

Self-Care Affirmation 4.4

I Can Feel Better

This affirmation helps you focus your mind on feeling better instead of on your illness.

===============

I Can Feel Better

Say this out loud 3 times:

"I can do whatever I focus my mind on.

If I can imagine it then I can do it.

Therefore, I can feel better if I focus my mind on feeling better."

===============

Self-Care Affirmation 4.5

I Am Thankful

This affirmation helps you remember all the things you have to be thankful for. One study showed gratitude improved happiness and health.

===============

I Am Thankful

Repeat the following out loud:

I am thankful for who I am.

I am thankful for what I have.

I am thankful for my family.

I am thankful for my friends.

I am thankful for my food.

I am thankful for my home.

I am thankful for my work.

I am thankful for my health.

I am thankful for my faith.

I am thankful for _____.

===============

Self-Care Affirmation 4.6

All Is Well

This affirmation helps you shift your mind and body into a safe place by repeating an exhale (which calms the sympathetic nervous system) and "All is well".

===============

All Is Well

A: Inhale through your nose as you slowly count to 4. 1-2-3-4.

B: Exhale through your mouth as you count to 8. 1-2-3-4-5-6-7-8.

C: Now silently say "All is well."

Repeat A) through C) for 4 breaths several times every day.

Notice what shifts in your mind and body when you do this.

=============

Self-Care Affirmation 4.7

It's Going to Be Alright

This affirmation helps you calm you fear or stress by reminding yourself that everything is going to be alright.

===============

It's Going to Be Alright

Whenever you feel worried, scared or stressed repeat this out loud 4 times:

"Everything is going to be alright."

Notice how you feel before and after doing this.

Print out an image that makes you smile such as a photo of a kitten and post it with this affirmation. Post this where you can see it to remind you.

===============

Self-Care Affirmation 4.8

I Feel Happy

This affirmation helps you feel better by tuning into the many things that make you feel happy. Use it whenever you notice you are feeling down.

===============

I Feel Happy

Read this out loud. I feel happy when:

I smile

I think thoughts that feel good

I help someone

I remember a happy time

I see family that I love

I do something I enjoy

I notice this moment

I complete a task

I am outside in nature

I meditate

I am thankful

(Add your own)

===============

Self-Care Affirmation 4.9

I Am Kind to Myself

This affirmation reminds you to be kind to yourself and to treat yourself well. Saying this out loud will help you actually be kind and treat yourself well when you notice you are being unkind to yourself.

===============

I am Kind to Myself

Say this out loud:

"I am kind to myself.

I treat myself well.

I speak kind words.

I replace unkind thoughts with kind thoughts.

I replace unkind self-talk with kind self-talk."

Practice doing it.

===============

Self-Care Affirmation 4.10

Things I Say To Myself

This affirmation helps you remember you are good enough, kind and caring and that you can allow yourself to feel well. This helps you interrupt negative self-talk so use it whenever you notice yourself doing it.

===============

Things I Say to Myself

Say this out loud:

"I am good enough

I believe in myself

I am kind

I am caring

I am brave

I allow myself to feel well"

===============

Self-Care Affirmation 4.11

I Am Safe

This affirmation encourages you to remember a time or situation when you felt completely safe and to go there in your mind whenever you need to. This helps your mind and body turn down your stress response.

===============

I Am Safe

Think of a time when you felt completely safe or imagine a situation where you feel safe.

Use this memory or image to create a safe haven in your mind.

Go there in your mind whenever you need to as you repeat out loud:

"I am safe."

===============

Self-Care Affirmation 4.12

I Love Myself

This affirmation helps you practice saying "I love you" out loud to yourself while looking in a mirror. Be mindful to silence your inner critic.

===============

I Love Myself

Look in the mirror.

Look at your face.

Smile.

Say this out loud 3 times:

"I love you 'your name'."

Notice how you feel after you do this.

Keep doing this until you can really feel the love you have for yourself without judgement.

===============

Self-Care Affirmation 4.13

My Why

Studies show that having a compelling reason to get well can be a powerful motivator in your healing journey. Use this affirmation to get in touch with, and remind yourself, of yours. This affirmation operationalizes the work you did in <u>Skill 3.10 My Reasons</u>.

=================

My Why

Repeat out loud several times daily:

"I want to be alive and well because:

(Fill in with your list, which may change periodically.)"

Allow yourself to feel and gently accept the emotions that arise while doing this.

=================

Radical Self-Care When You Are Ill Worksheet

Download a free version of this worksheet online at https://thebrainlady.com/radical-self-care-downloads/ and print it out or save it as a document in your word processor. Use it as a template and expand it to insert and add to your answers each time you do a skill that directs you to write them down. You will create a valuable resource to help you stay focused on your healing journey. Review what you wrote regularly.

EMOTIONAL WELL-BEING

1.1 My HEALING INTENTION is:

1.2 I will eliminate or CHANGE THESE STRESSORS:

1.3 I will CHANGE THE CHANNEL in my mind to watch these channels that feel good to watch:

1.4 This will be DIFFERENT WHEN I AM WELL:

1.5 Things that NEED TO CHANGE:

PHYSICAL WELL-BEING

2.1 Questions I will ASK MY DOCTOR:

2.3 My HEALING TEAM members (with contact information) will include:

2.5 This is how I will CHANGE MY DIET to heal:

2.6 I feel best when I get ___hours of sleep.

2.6 I will GO TO BED at: ______ and get up at: _______.

2.7 This is the EXERCISE I will do and when I will do it:

2.9 I will set these MINDFUL LIMITS to prevent getting exhausted:

MIND-BODY-SPIRIT WELL-BEING

3.1 I BELIEVE:

3.3 I need HELP with:

3.3 I will ask these people for HELP when I need it:

3.5 Here is my HEALING PRAYER:

3.8 GUIDANCE I received:

3.9: I received this from LOVED ONES in spirit:

3.10 MY REASONS to be well and alive:

3.11 INTUITION I received:

3.12 This is how I will BE OF SERVICE:

3.13 My current SOCIAL SUPPORT SYSTEM:

3.13 This is how I will expand my SOCIAL SUPPORT:

About the Author

Debra Burdick, LCSW is an international expert on Mindfulness and ADHD, and a best-selling, award winning author.

She teaches professionals, groups and individuals how to integrate mindfulness into their lives and work. She is a pioneer in using mindfulness skills to improve mental and physical health. She first started creating and using skills in this book to turn down her pain and deal with a painful chronic illness, now thankfully healed.

Visit: www.TheBrainLady.com for more information and resources.

References

Adams, R. (2010). Improving health outcomes with better patient understanding and education, *Risk Management and Healthcare Policy*, 3:61-72.

Amen, Daniel. (2015). *Change Your Brain Change Your Life*. (Revised and Expanded). Harmony.

Benson, H. (2000). *The Relaxation Response*. (Updated ed.). William Morrow Paperbacks.

Benson, H. M.D. and Friedman, R. Ph.D. (1996). *Harnessing the Power of the Placebo Effect and Renaming It "Remembered Wellness"*. Annual Review of Medicine. 47:1,193-199

Burdick, D. (2013. *Mindfulness Skills for Clinicians and Clients*. PESI, Eau Claire, WI.

Boelens PA, Reeves RR, Replogle WH, Koenig HG. (2009). A randomized trial of the effect of prayer on depression and anxiety. *Int J Psychiatry Med*. 39(4):377-92.

Cousins, N. (1979). Anatomy of an illness as perceived by the patient: reflections on healing and regeneration. New York: Norton.

Fehmi, L. (2010). *Dissolving pain: Simple brain training exercises for overcoming pain.* Boston: Trumpeter Books.

Jacobsen, E. (1929). *Progressive Relaxation*. Univ. Of Chicago Press, Oxford.

Kabat-Zinn J. (2003). Mindfulness-based interventions in context: Past, present, and future. *Clinical Psychology: Science and Practice*. 10:144–156.

Kabat-Zinn J. 2013. Using the wisdom of your body and mind to face stress, pain, and illness. *Full Catastrophe Living. (Rev Ed)*. New York, NY: Bantam Books.

Moorijani, Anita (2012). *Dying to be Me*. Hay House, Australia.

Oarga, C., Stavrova, O., & Fetchenhauer, D. (2015). When and why is helping others good for well-being? The role of belief in reciprocity and conformity to society's expectations. *European Journal of Social Psychology, 45*(2), 242–254.

Over, C., Sinatra, S, Zucher, M. (2014). *Earthing: The Most Important Health Discovery Ever!* Basic Health Publications, Inc., Laguna Beach, CA.

Ranganathan VK, Siemionow V, Liu JZ, Sahgal V, (2004).Yue GH. From mental power to muscle power--gaining strength by using the mind. *Neuropsychologia*. 42(7):944-56.

Schneiderman N, Ironson G, Siegel SD.(2015). Stress and health: psychological, behavioral, and biological determinants. *Annu Rev Clin Psychol*. 1:607-28.

Turner, K. (2014). *Radical Remission: Surviving Cancer Against All Odds, Harper Collins Publishing*, New York, NY.

Uchino, B., Bowen, K., Kent de Grey, R., Mikel, J., Fisher, E., (2018). Social Support and Physical Health: Models, Mechanisms, and Opportunities, *Principles and Concepts of Behavioral Medicine*, 2018. ISBN : 978-0-387-93825-7

Watson, N. F., Badr, M. S., Belenky, G., Bliwise, D. L., Buxton, O. M., Buysse, D., Dinges, D. F., Gangwisch, J., Grandner, M. A., Kushida, C., Malhotra, R. K., Martin, J. L., Patel, S. R., Quan, S. F., & Tasali, E. (2015).

Recommended amount of sleep for a healthy adult: A joint consensus statement of the American Academy of Sleep Medicine and Sleep Research Society. *Journal of Clinical Sleep Medicine*, *11*(06), 591–592. https://doi.org/10.5664/jcsm.4758

van de Kolk, B. (2014). *The Body Keeps the Score: Brain, Mind and Body in the Healing of Trauma*, Penguin Books.

www.TheBrainLady.com

ALSO BY AWARD-WINNING, BEST-SELLING AUTHOR

DEBRA BURDICK

Radical Self-Care When You Are Ill – Card Deck

Mindfulness Skills Workbook for Clinicians and Clients –

#1 best seller on amazon

Mindfulness for Kids with ADHD

Mindfulness Skills for Kids Card Deck and Card Games

Mindfulness for Teens with ADHD

ADHD: Non-Medication Treatments and Skills for Children and Teens   Benjamin Franklin GOLD award in Psychology

Mindfulness Skills Workbook for Kids and Teens

Meditations for Concentration CD/mp3

Mindfulness Toolkit CD/mp3

Mindfulness Toolkit for Kids mp3

Mindfulness: Basics and Beyond Teletraining

Transforming Stress Teletraining

Meditation for Sleep